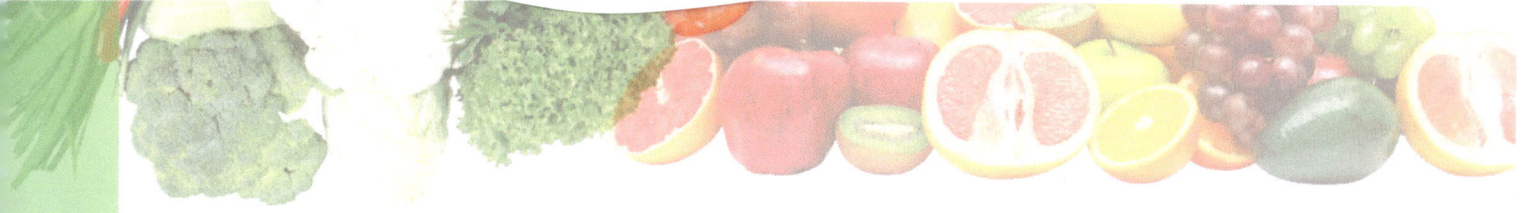

"MY GUT, GOT THE GUTS TO DEAL WITH ME BECAUSE OF MY POOR DIETARY HABITS."

QUOTE BY
MRS NANCY OGBOI
20TH OCTOBER 2018.

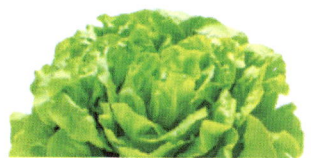

DISCLAIMER

The information provided in this juice recipe book is intended for general informational purposes only. The recipes, contained herein are not intended to be a substitute for professional medical advice, diagnosis, or treatment. Always seek the advice of your physician or other qualified health provider with any questions you may have regarding a medical condition or dietary needs.

Individuals with specific health concerns, allergies, dietary restrictions, or medical conditions should consult with a healthcare professional before making any dietary changes or consuming any of the juices included in this recipe book.

Every effort has been made to ensure that the information and recipes provided in this book are accurate and up to date at the time of publication.

By using this recipe book, you acknowledge that you have read, understood, and agree to abide by this disclaimer.
If you do not agree to these terms, please refrain from using this book.

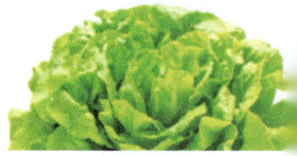

JUICING FOR GENERAL HEALTH WELLNESS

Juicing is when fresh vegetables are fed through a juicer, not a blender. The juicer separates the juice from the pulp and concentrates all the vegetable nutrients in an easily digestible juice. This means that the juice can deliver much more nutrition to your cells quicker and with much less energy than disgesting whole food.

These juices prevent diseases and even reverse them.
For these juice recipes, you will need a high-quality juicer. Juicers come in many shapes and sizes and use various extraction mechanisms.

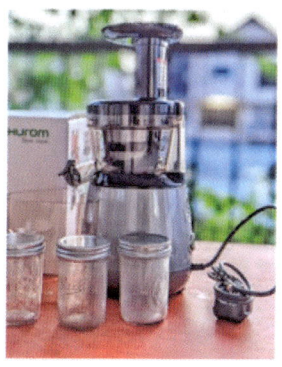

Hurom Slow Juicer Storage Container
Available to order.
 +234 705 290 0990

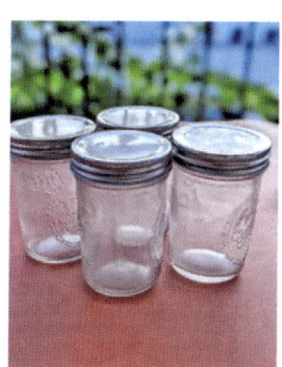

The slower the speed, the better. They slowly crush the vegetables without degrading the juice with heat and air, thereby minimising loss of enzyme or nutrition.
Whereas high speed Juicers draw air and heat into the juicing mechanism destroying enzymes .

If you're ready to experience the healing power of these stress-free recipes, you can conveniently shop the juicer and begin your transformative journey towards vibrant health.

INTRODUCTION TO MY JUICE RECIPE BOOK

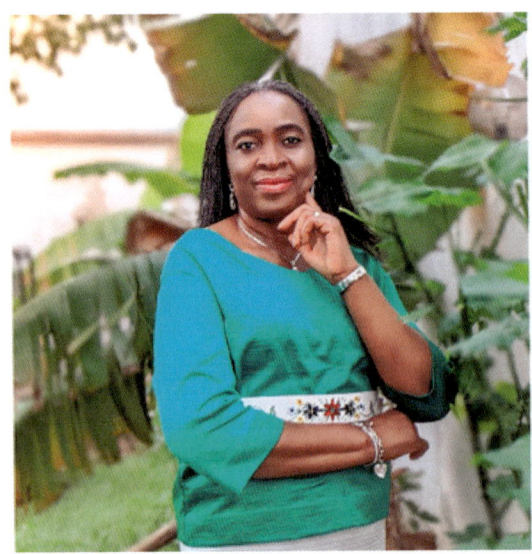

Congratulations on making a decision to take charge of your health. You really do not have to wait until you are diagnosed with an aliment or illness before you switch to a "Healthy lifestyle"
This sounds simple. It's often not easy. But cheaper than illness.
I have been there before.

In 2018, I was diagnosed with cancer. I went through chemotherapy and combined it with vegetable juicing throughout the eight sessions.

I am not a medical doctor, but I am sharing the experience of dealing mostly with juicing, which helped me through my journey of recovery and healing. My juicing experience has helped many people, including children, who have different kinds of ailment that I am coaching and mentoring.

My goal is to empower you to experience vibrant health by sharing the juice recipes that have been integral to my own healing journey.

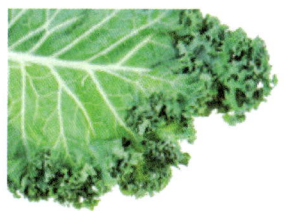

SIMPLE RECIPES

GREEN DELIGHT

- ½ Handful of spinach
- 1 Green apple
- ½ Cucumber
- 1" Ginger

LOCAL VITALITY

- 5 Utazi leaves
- 1 Oziza leaf
- 10 Scent leaves
- 1 Medium cucumber
- ½ Lemon

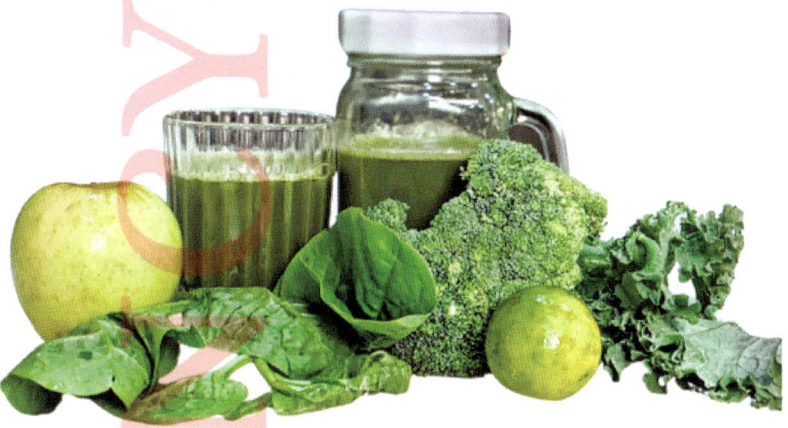

SWEET GREEN

- 1 Cucumber
- 1 Handful spinach
- 1 Green apple
- 1 Lime juice

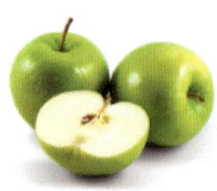

HEALTH BOOSTER

- 1 Handful Ewedu
- 5 Leaves of Hospital too far (Chaya)
- 3 Big Miracle leaves
- 4 Celery stalks
- 1" Ginger

JOYOUS

- 1 Handful Kale
- 1 Handful Parsley
- 1 Handful Spinach
- 1 Small green apple
- ½ Green Bell Pepper

GREEN JUICE

- 1 Cucumber
- 1 Handful of ugwu leaf
- 1 Green apple
- 5 Kale leaves
- 3 Celery stalks
- 1" Ginger

KIDNEY FRIENDLY

- 5 Kale leaves
- ½ Handful of parsley
- 3 Celery stalks [without leaves]
- ½ Cucumber
- 1" Ginger
- 1 Lime

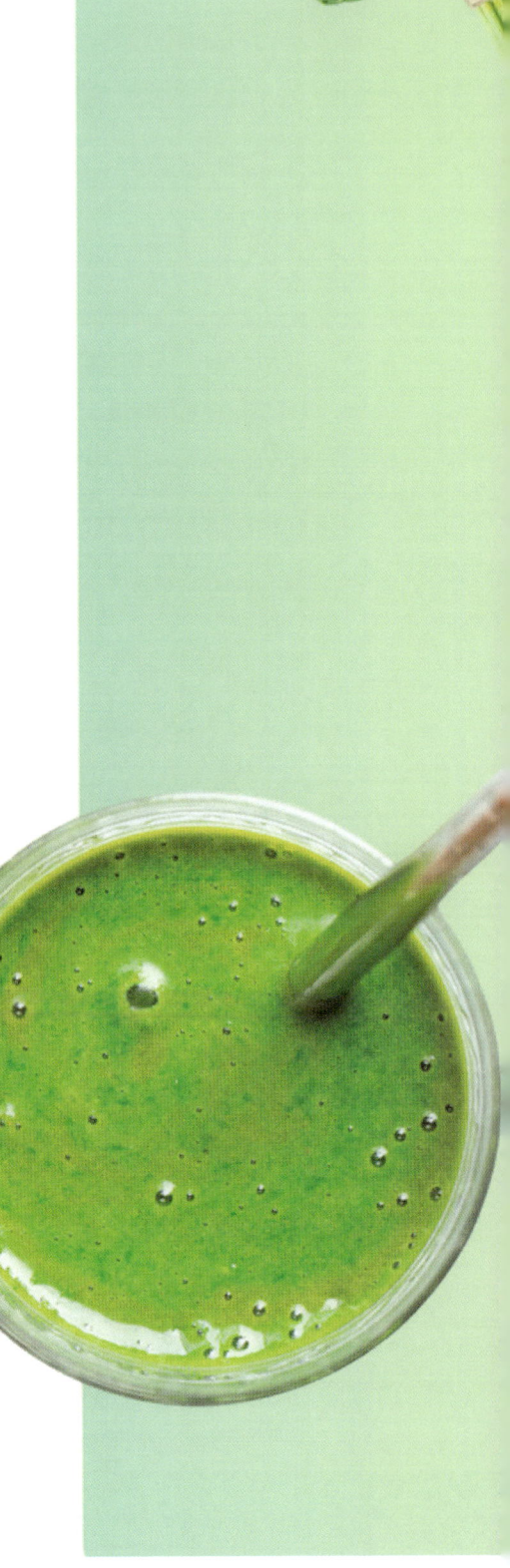

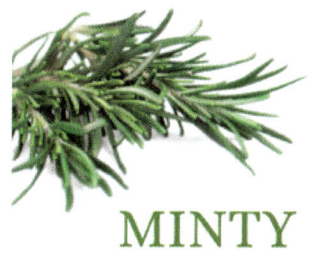

MINTY

- 1 Handful of mint leaf
- 1 Cucumber
- ½ Lemon
- 1" Ginger

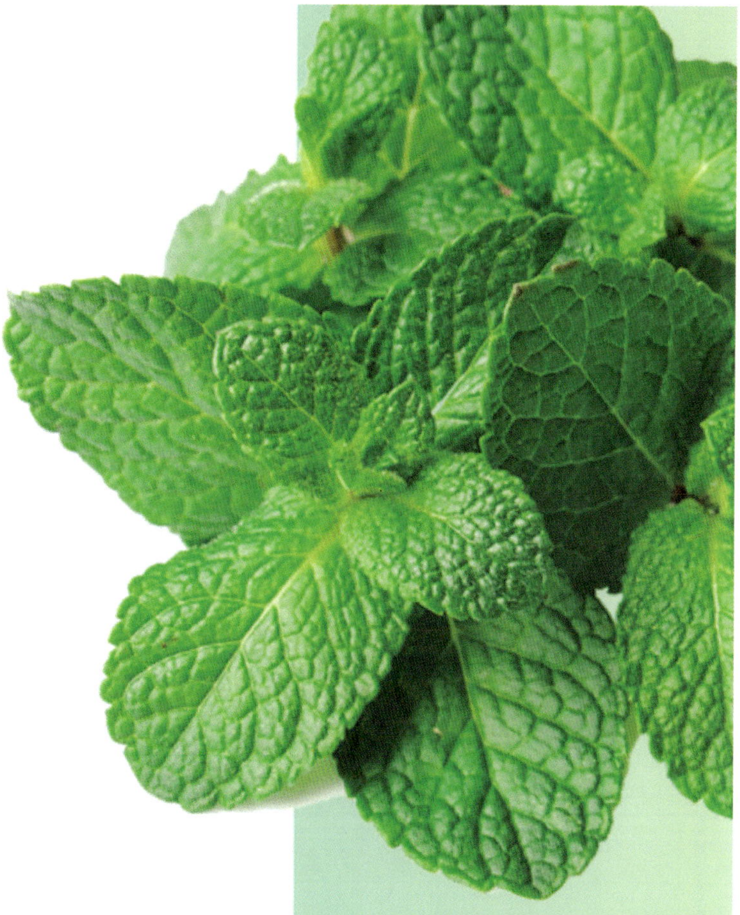

BITTER GALL

- 10 Bitter leaf
- 5 Utazi leaves
- 1 Handful Garden egg leaf
- 1 Bitter Kola
- 1 Lime

POWER UP

- 2 Celery stalk
- 3 Kale leaves
- ½ Handful Ewedu
- ½ Handful Parsley
- ½ Handful Coriander
- 3 Big Miracle leaves
- 1/3 Cucumber
- ½ Lemon

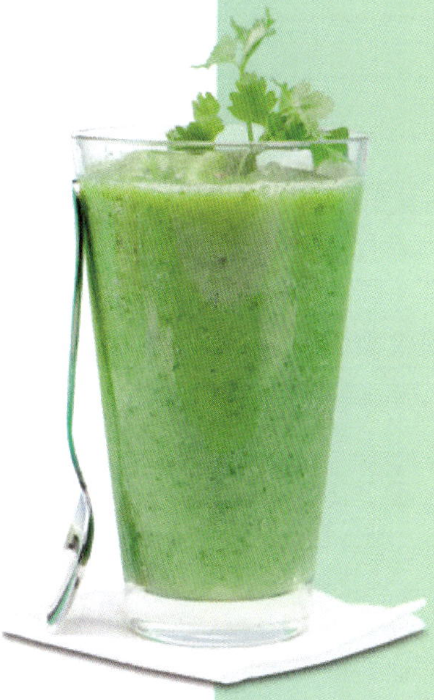

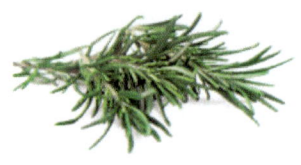

BOUNTIFUL
- 1 Handful of Ewedu
- ½ Medium Cucumber
- 1 Handful Hospital too far
- 1" Ginger

DETOX TEA
- ½ Medium sized Fennel
- 3 Celery stalks
- 1" Ginger
- 1 Lime

GREEN REVITALIZER
- 1 Handful of Ugwu
- ½ Medium Cucumber
- 2 Small Green apples

ENERGIZER
- 3 Celery stalks
- 5 Kale leaves
- ½ Handful of Spinach
- ½ Lemon
- 1 Medium Cucumber

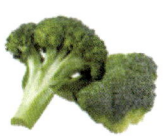

EMERALD BOOST

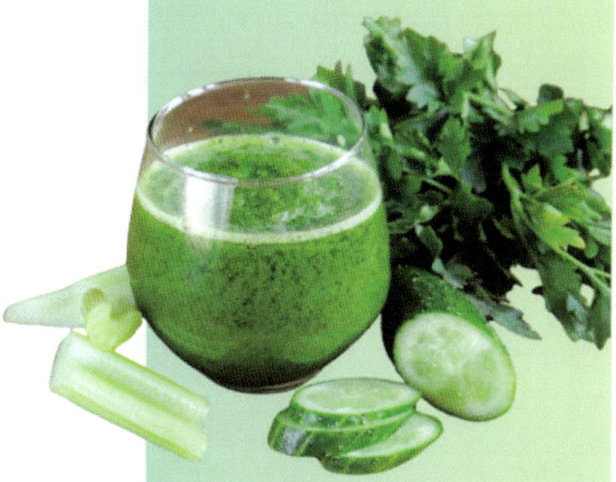

- 1 Handful of Parsley
- 1 Handful Coriander
- Small fresh Rosemary
- Small fresh Thyme
- Small fresh Oregano
- 1 Lime
- ½ Medium Cucumber
- Small fresh Basil

GALL CLEANSE

- 1½ Handful of Mint leaves
- ¼ Broccoli
- 1 Medium Cucumber
- 10 Mustard leaves
- 1 Lime

GREEN SPLASH

- 1 Handful of Rocket Arugula
- 1 Handful Gardenegg leaves
- 1 Medium Cucumber
- 1" Ginger

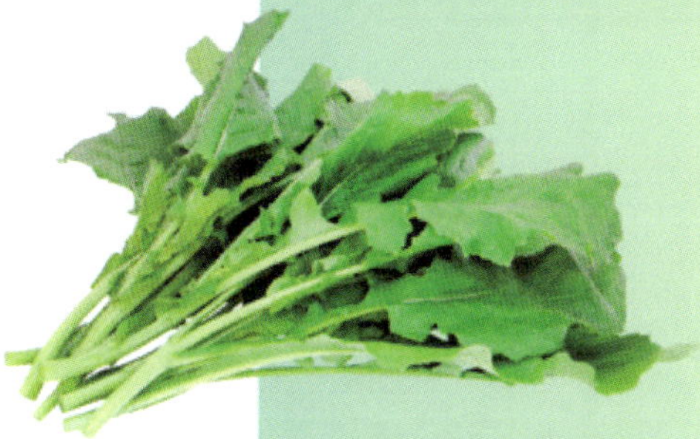

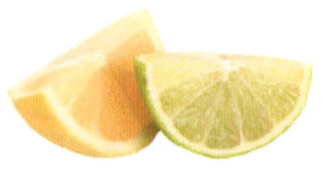
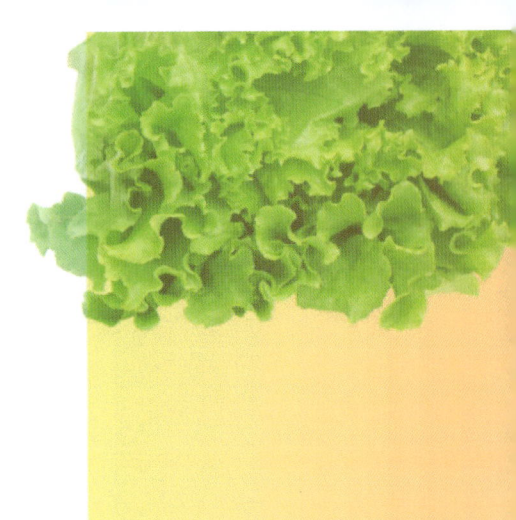

GOLDEN JUICE

- ½ of a big mango no skin
- 1 Yellow bell pepper
- 1 Cucumber
- 1 Turmeric + a pinch of black pepper
- 1" Ginger

YELLOW MAGIC

- 1 Turmeric + a pinch of black pepper
- 1" Ginger
- ½ Lemon
- 1 Yellow bell pepper
- ½ Medium pineapple

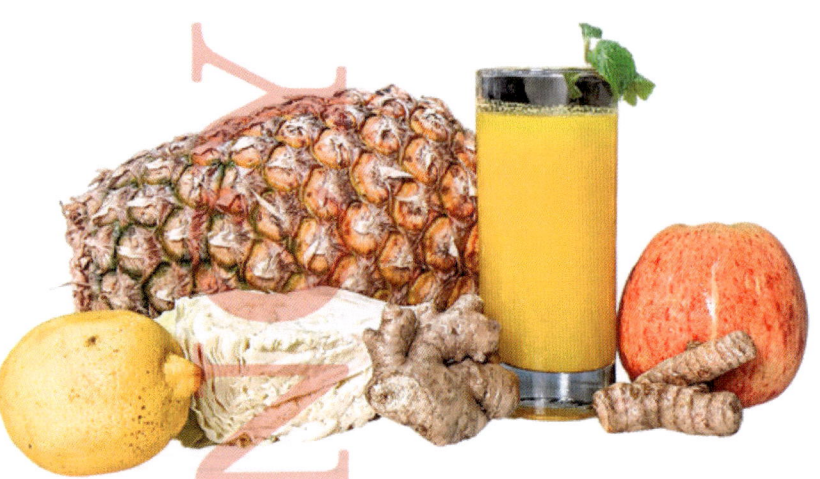

GOODNESS

- 1/3 Medium broccoli
- ¼ Medium pineapple
- 5 Kale leaves
- 1 English pear

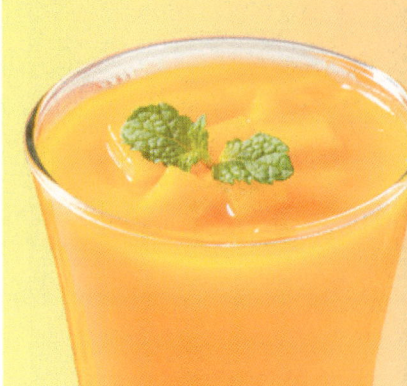

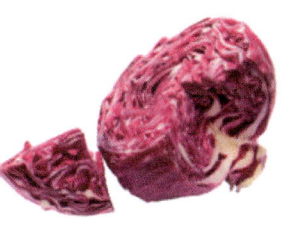

PURPLE JUICE

- ¼ Medium Purple cabbage
- 1 Handful of Seedless grapes
- 1 Red apple

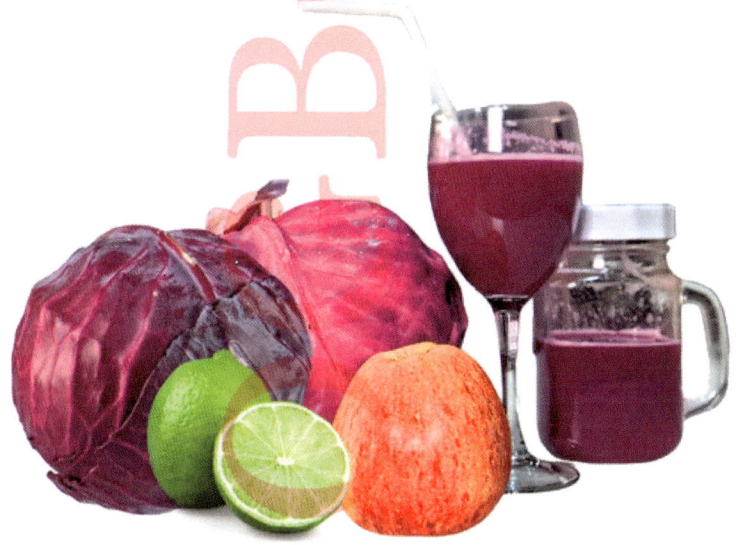

ROYAL FLUSH

- 1 Lime
- ½ Cucumber
- 1 Orange
- 1/8 Medium Purple cabbage
- 1 Stalk of Fennel chopped
- 3 Celery stalks
- ¼ Medium broccoli

GUT FRIENDLY

- ¼ Medium Pineapple
- ½ Red Beetroot
- 1" Ginger

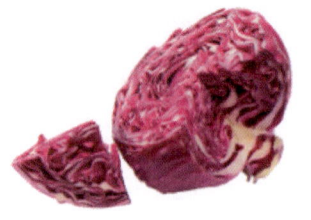

LAVENDER

- ¼ Medium Purple cabbage
- 5 Miracle leaves
- 3 Utazi leaves
- ¼ Medium Cucumber
- 1" Ginger

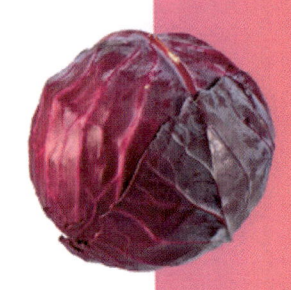
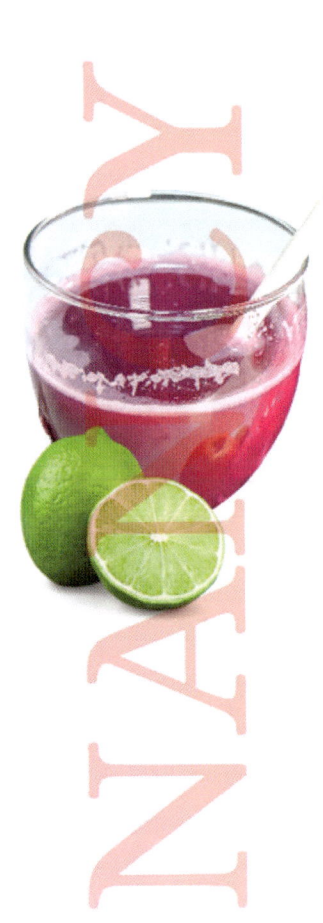
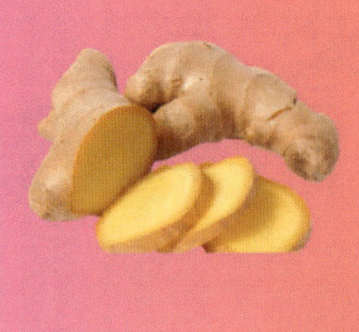

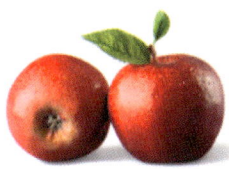

STRAWBERRY BLISS

- 10 Strawberries
- 4 Fresh tomatoes
- 1 Cup chopped watermelon
- Few basil leaves

RUBY DELIGHT

- 1 Beetroot
- 3 Medium carrots
- 5 Kale leaves
- 1 Small red apple
- 1" Ginger

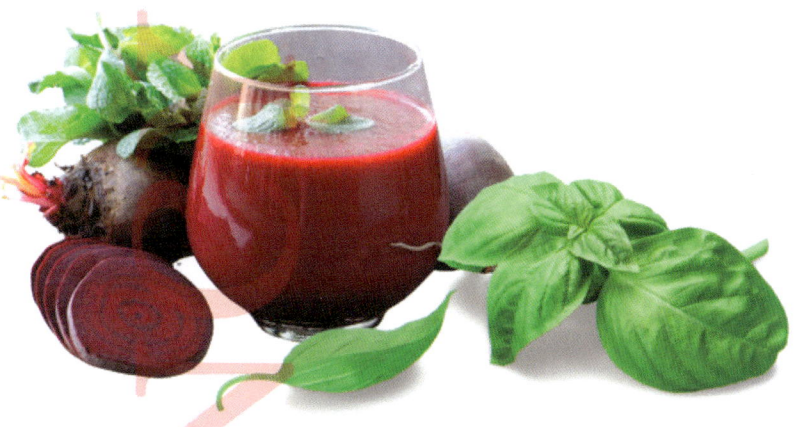

CELL REFRESHER

- 2 Apples
- 1 Beetroot
- 1 Cup spinach
- Few mint leaves

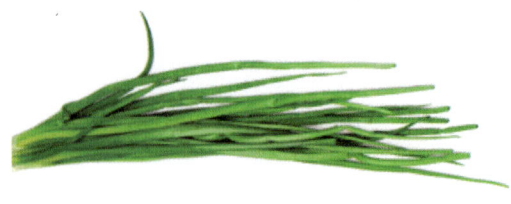

SPICY STEW

- 5 Fresh tomatoes
- 1 Red bell pepper
- 1 Habanero pepper
- 1 small Leek stalk
- 3 Spring onion
- Few fresh rosemary leaves
- Few fresh thyme leaves
- ½ Handful Parsley
- 1" Ginger
- 3 Cloves garlic

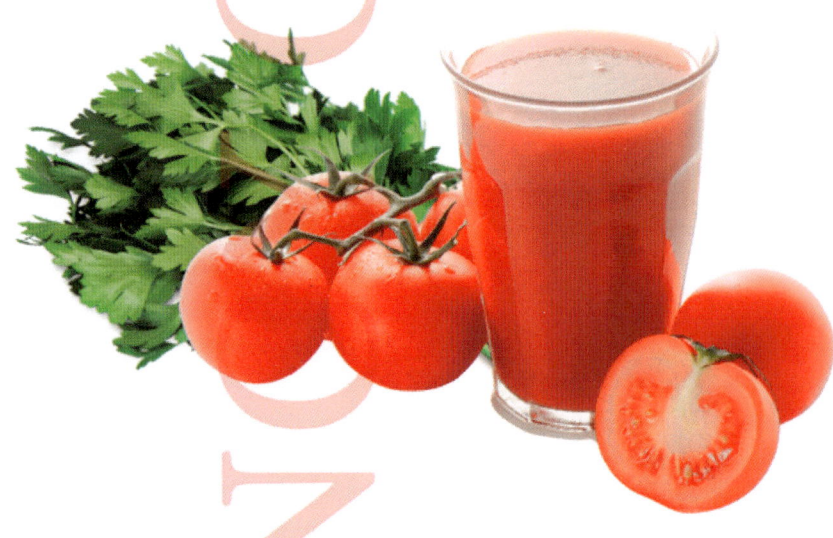

BLOOD TONIC

- ½ Beetroot
- ½ Handful of ugwu leaf
- ½ Handful of gardern egg leaf
- ½ Lemon
- 1/3 Cucumber

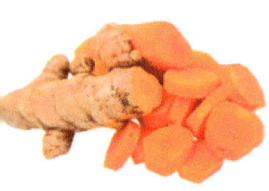

NUTRI- JUICE

- 15 Carrots
- 1 Orange
- 1 Lemon
- 1" Ginger

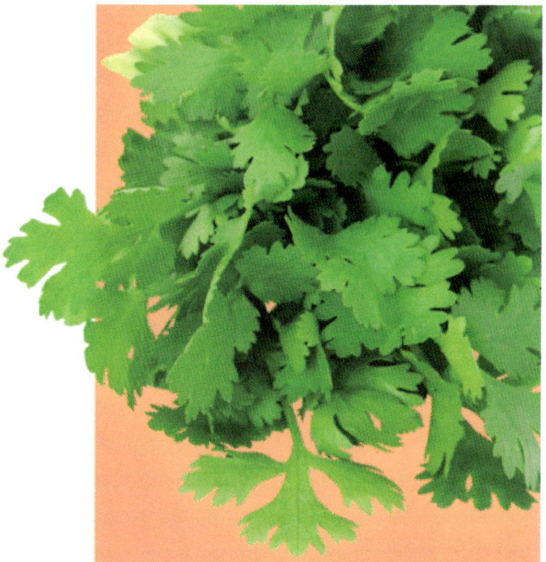

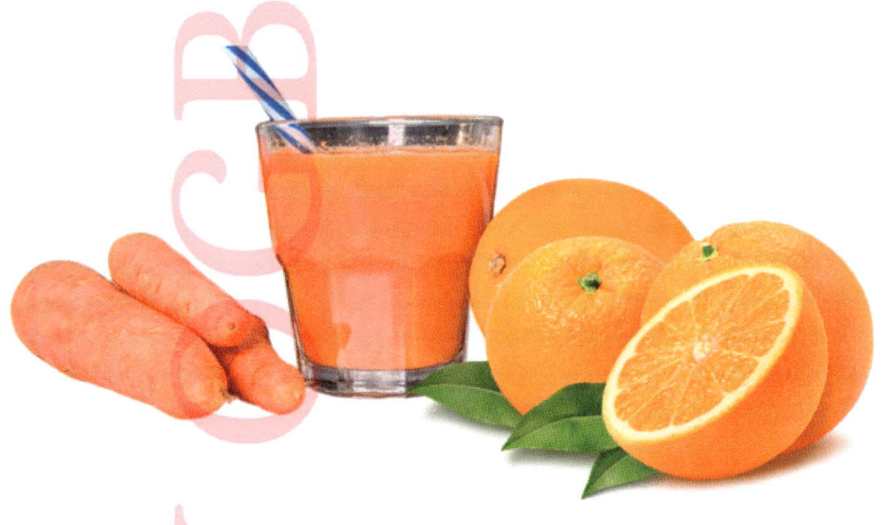

PURE CARROT JUICE

- 10 Medium Carrot
- ½ Lemon

GOLDEN GLOW

- 1 Orange
- 10 Carrots
- 1 Orange Bell pepper
- 1 Lemon
- ½ Handful of Mint

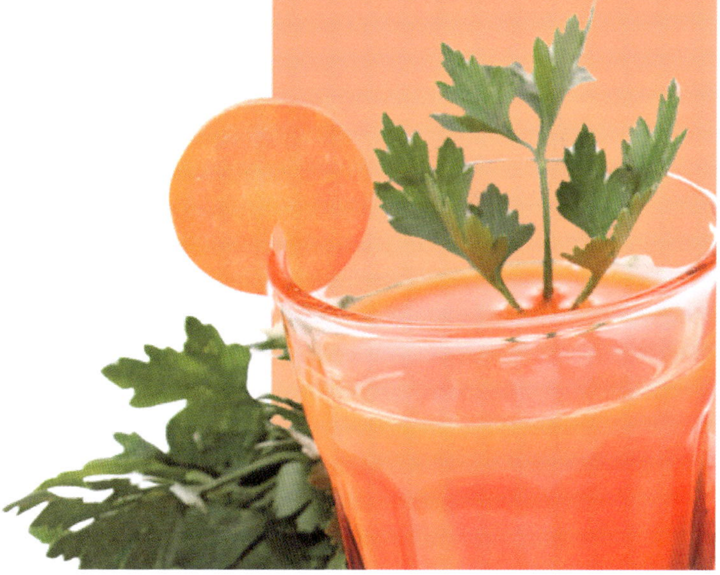

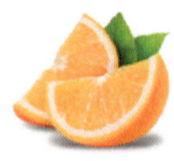

CARROT MAGIC

- 1 English Pear
- 3 Carrots
- ¼ Medium Cabbage
- 1 Handful Kale
- 1 Lemon with skin

PARADISE

- 10 Carrots
- ½ Beetroot
- ½ Cucumber
- 1" Ginger

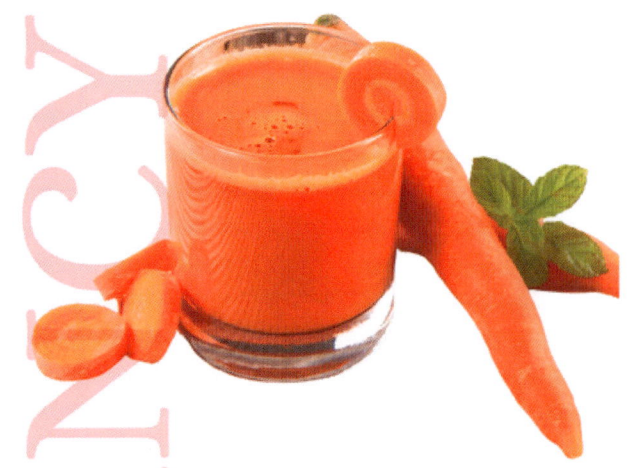

FAT BLAST

- 1 Big grapefruit
- 3 Cloves of garlic
- 1 Lemon with skin

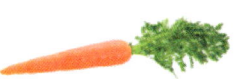

GOLDEN VITALITY

- 5 Medium Carrots
- 1 Bunch of Bok choy
- 1 Handful Ugwu leaves
- 1 Small Pomegranate seeds

REJOICE

- 5 Medium Carrots
- 1 Handful Dandelion
- ½ Lemon
- 2 Big leaves of Hospital too far

TONIC ELIXIR

- 5 Medium Carrots
- 1 Handful fresh Spring beans
- ½ Medium Cucumber
- ½ Handful Parsley

SUNSET BLISS

- 5 Medium Carrots
- ½ Medium Cucumber
- ½ Medium Broccoli
- ½ Handful Dill

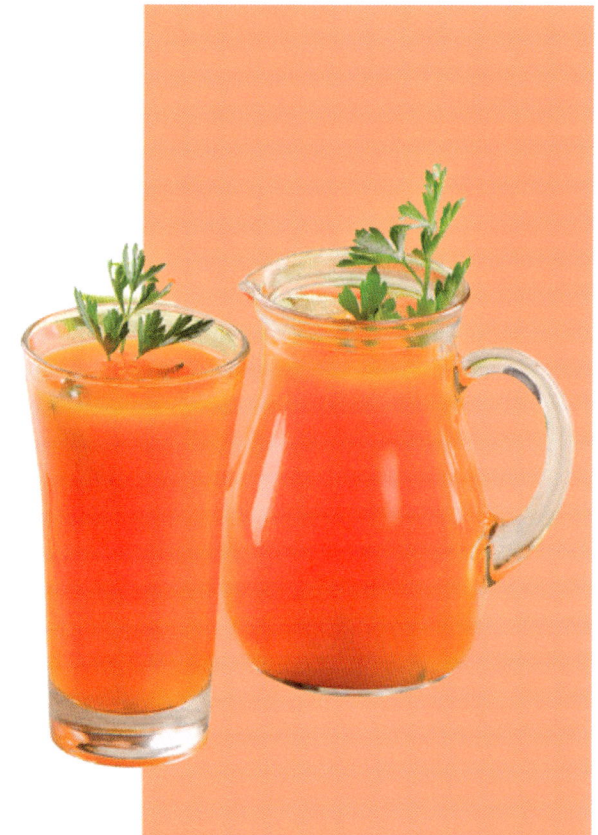

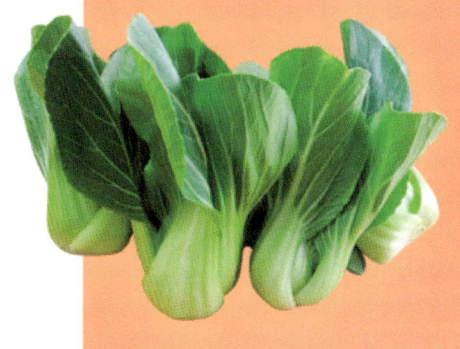

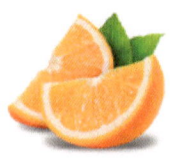

ANTIOXIDANT

- 5 Medium carrots
- 1 Bunch of Lettuce
- ½ Medium Cucumber
- 3 Celery

CELL CLEANSE

- 5 Medium carrots
- 1 Handful Spring beans
- 1 Green Apple
- 1 Bunch Lettuce

RADIANT SPLASH

- 5 Medium carrots
- ¼ Medium Cabbage
- 1 Handful Dandelion leaves
- 1 Lemon

CARROT SHAKE

- 5 Medium carrots
- 1 Small bunch of Bok choy
- 10 Gardern egg leaves
- ½ Medium Cucumber

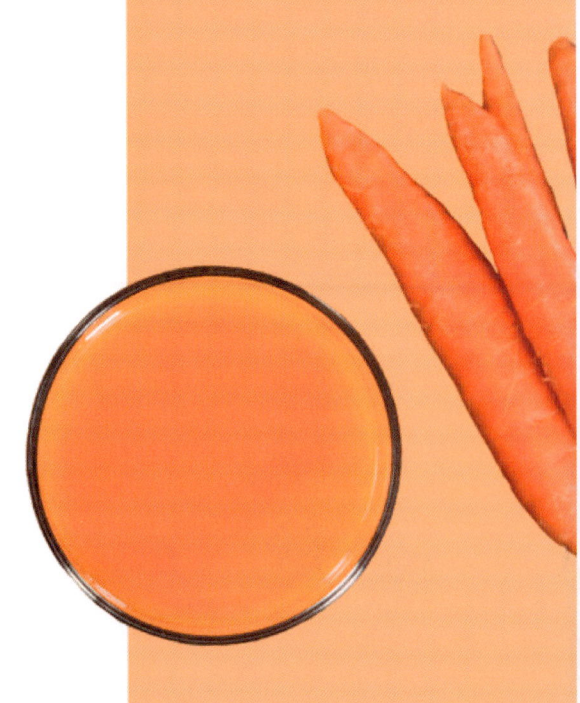

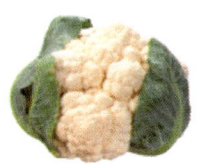

FAT BELLY BURNER

- 1 Lemon or 1 Lime
- 1 Medium Cucumber
- 1" Ginger
- ¼ Grapefruit
- ¼ Cup Blueberry
- ¼ Medium Pineapple
- ½ Cup Spinach
- 2 Celery stalks
- ½ Handful Parsley
- 1 Tbsp Apple cider vinegar

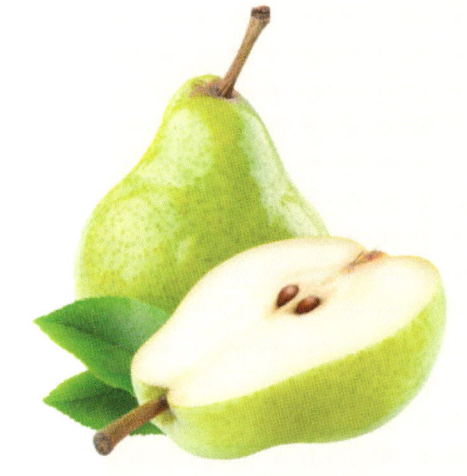

SUNSHINE JUICE

- 1 Grapefruit
- 1 Cucumber
- 1 Green apple
- ½ Beets
- 1" Ginger

COLON DETOX

- ½ Pineapple
- 1 Celery
- 1 Cucumber
- 1" Ginger

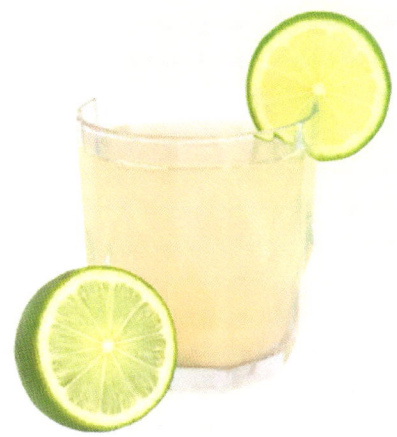

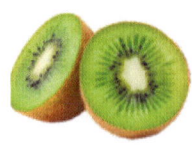

RENEWAL

- 1 Celery stalk
- 1 Lemon

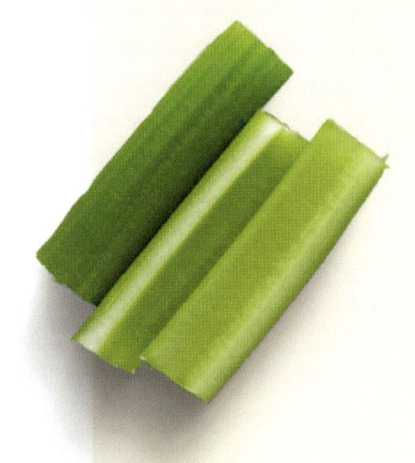

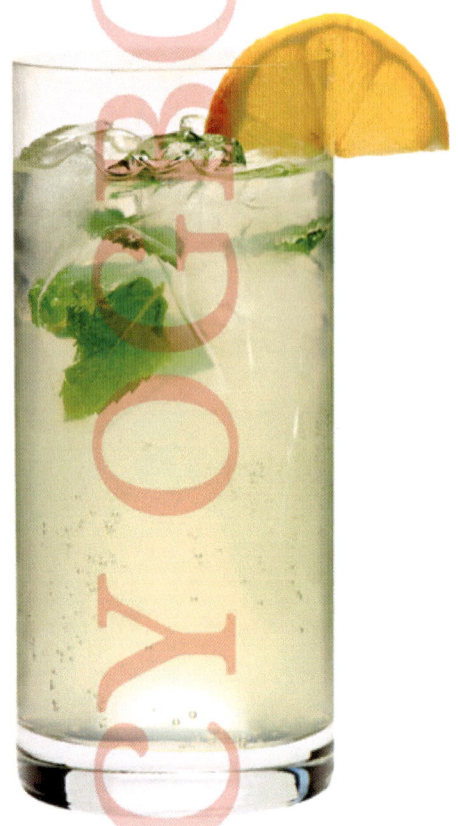

NUTRIENT NECTAR

- 3 Stalks of Celery
- 1 Small Green apple
- 1 Lemon
- 1" Ginger

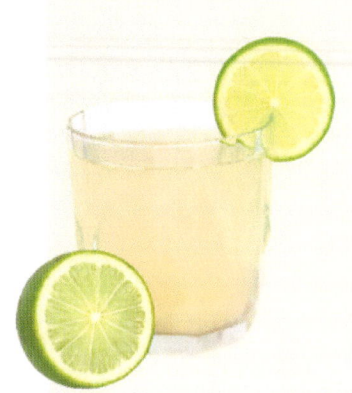

WONDER BLEND

- 1 Cup of Fresh Coconut water
- 1 Medium Cucumber
- 1 Green apple
- ¼ Medium Cabbage

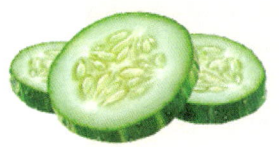

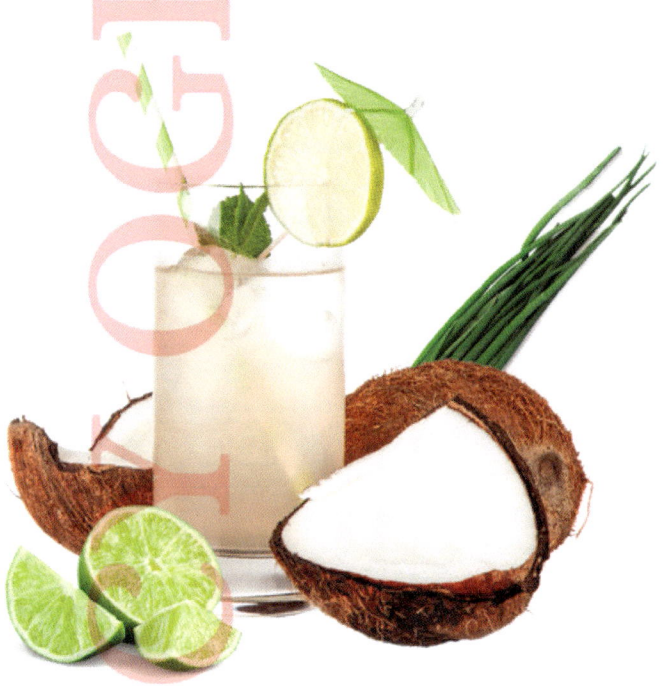

HARMONY

- 1 Cucumber
- 1 Grape
- 1 English pear
- 1 Kiwi
- ½ Handful of Mint

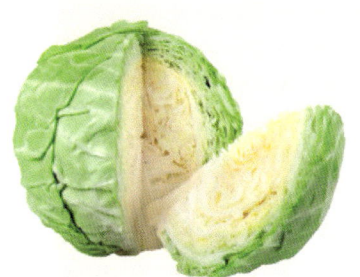

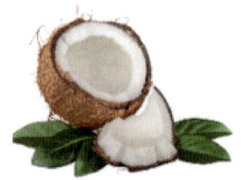

LIFE

- 1 big Turmeric+ a pinch of black pepper
- 1 Red pepper
- 3 Celery stalks
- 1 Green apple
- 1" Ginger

WELLNESS

- 1 Lime
- ½ Cucumber
- 1 Orange
- 1/8 medium Cabbage
- 1 stalk of Fennel chopped
- 3 Celery stalks
- 1/4 medium broccoli

HEART MIRACLE

- 1 cup of fresh Coconut water
- 1 Pomegranate
- ½ Beetroot
- ½ Lemon

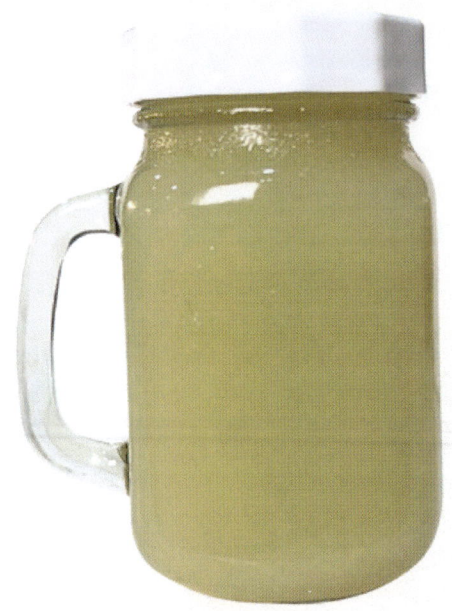

NOTE:
For special specific treatment, book a chat.

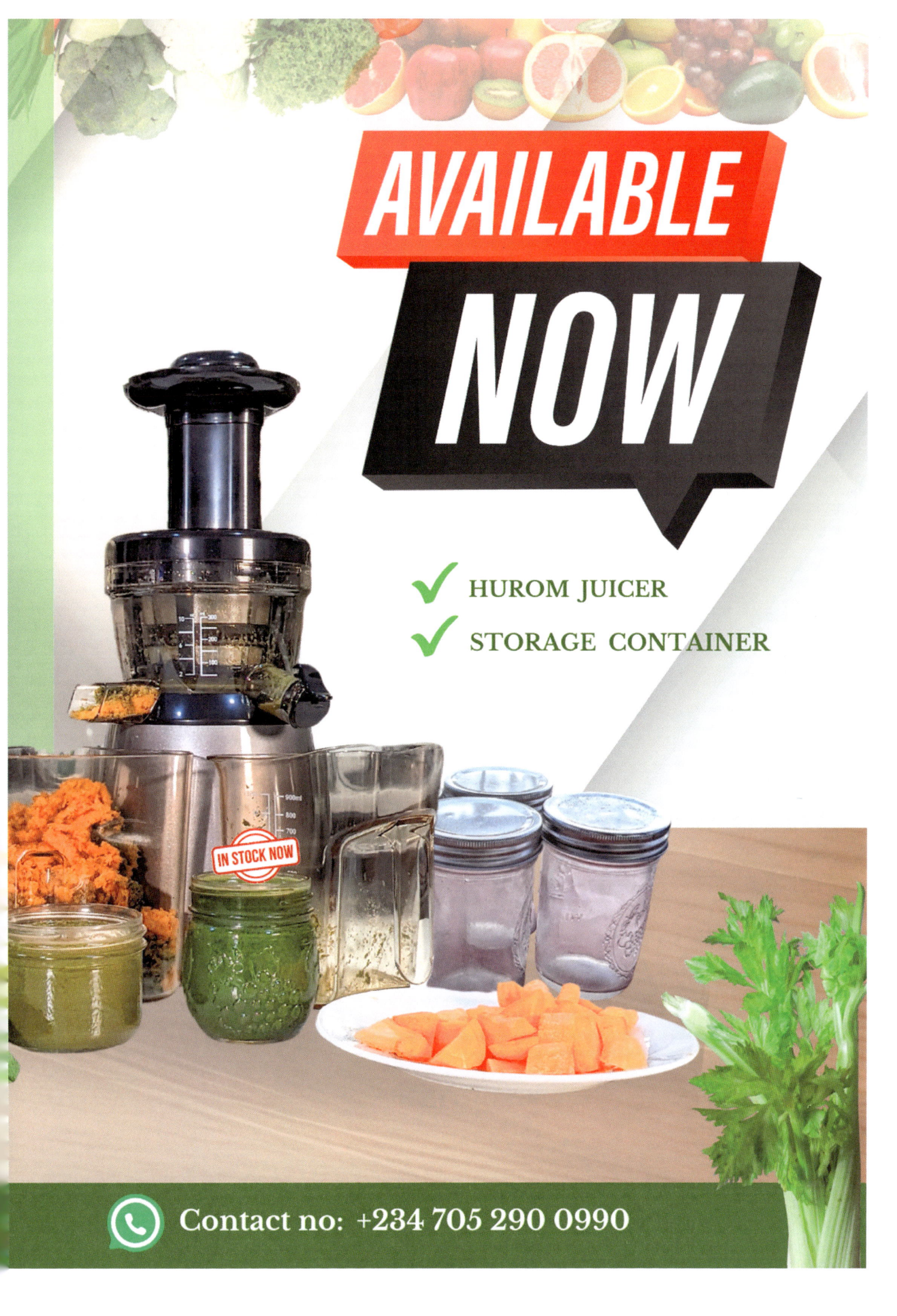

ACKNOWLEDGEMENT

I am filled with profound gratitude to Almighty God.
It has been an honor to embark on this journey of creation, one filled with passion, dedication, and a deep-seated commitment to fostering wellness.

To each and every one of you who has chosen to explore the pages of this book, I extend my heartfelt thanks. Your support and encouragement have been the driving force behind this endeavor, propelling me forward even in moments of doubt.

To my family, friends, and mentors, your unwavering belief in me has been a guiding light throughout this journey. Your encouragement, wisdom, and love have infused every page of this book with warmth and authenticity.

I extend my deepest appreciation to you, dear reader, for allowing me to share my passion for health and wellness with you. As you explore the recipes within these pages, it is my sincere wish they serve as a catalyst for positive change in your life, that it brings you joy, healing, nourishment, fulfillment, and not only years to your life also life to your years.

With gratitude and warmest regards,

Nancy Ogboi

© 2024

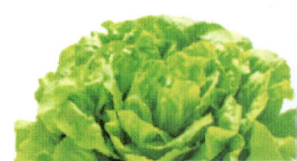

Printed in Great Britain
by Amazon